HOMEOPATHY FOR BIRTHING:

A simplified guide for mothers, midwives and other professionals

By Jana Shiloh, M.A.

2nd Edition

Rocky Mountain Press
Sedona, AZ

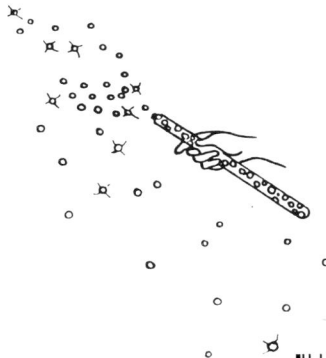

HOMEOPATHY FOR BIRTHING:

A simplified guide for mothers, midwives and other professionals

By Jana Shiloh, M.A.

Published by: Rocky Mountain Press
                     P.O. Box 10265
                     Sedona, AZ 86336
                     602-282-9362

Copyright 1990 and 1991 by Jana Shiloh
First Printing 1990
Second Printing 1991, revised
Printed in the United States of America

ISBN 0-9619203-2-7: $10.95 Softcover

Cover art and design by Linda Bruce
Text art by Sunshower

Table of Contents

REMEDIES

The following remedies are discussed for all aspects of birthing:

Aconite	Coffea	Nat Mur
Antemonium Tart	Gelsemium	Nux Moschata
Apis	Gossypium	Nux Vomica
Arnica	Hamamalis	Phosphorus
Belladonna	Hypericum	Platina
Bryonia	Ignatia	Pulsatilla
Calcarea Carbonicum	Ipecac	Pyrogenum
Cantharis	Kali Carbonicum	Ruta
Carbo Vegetabilas	Kreosotum	Sabina
Caulophllum	Lac Canninum	Secale
Chamomile	Lachesis	Sepia
China	Laurocerasus	
Cicuta	Lycopodium	
Cimicifuga	Magnesium Phos.	

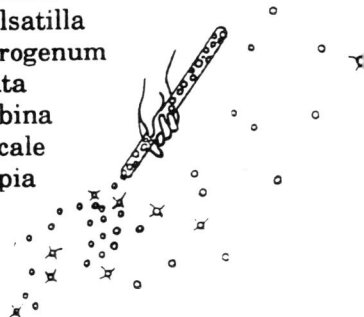

Bare Minimum First Aid Remedies For Birthing

Although any remedy needed in a specific situation is essential, the following are bare minimum remedies for *anyone's* birth:

1. Arnica — For physical injury: Used before and after the birth for the mother, and after the birth if there has been physical injury to the infant.
2. Aconite — For birth trauma: Used for the infant or panic for the mother.
3. Hypericum: Laceration of the perineum, or injury to the coccyx.
4. Staphysagria: Episiotomy. Problems with healing of any incision (ie. caesarian).
5. Antimonium Tart: Rattling mucus in the infant's lungs.
6. Cimicifuga: Used in low potency (12C or 30C) to induce slow labors.
7. Caulophyllum: Used in low potency (12C or 30C) to induce slow labors.

Please read about the above remedies in this book.

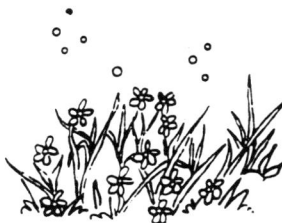

INTRODUCTION

This work was inspired by a desire to see midwives and other health professionals use homeopathy in their practice. Admittedly, the scientific art of homeopathy is challenging, even to a homeopath. The need to consider all aspects of the individual before coming to the correct remedy makes selection complicated, and has discouraged most midwives from its use.

The fact is that in homeopathy, as opposed to most other modalities, we look for clues (symptoms) to form a picture. This includes the physical *and* the emotional levels. We then find ONE remedy whose "remedy picture" matches that of the patient. Dramatic and speedy results are noted when the correct remedy is given

This work is not original in that all of the information can be found in the works of J. Tyler Kent, W.A. Yingling, and Clarke's Materia Medica (see bibliography). Although I have had experience attending births, I am not a midwife; I am a homeopath. The purpose of this work however, is to make homeopathy more accessible for those interested in using it for birthing and other problems in obstetrics. In order to do this, I have arranged the material in a form as to make remedy selection easier.

The keynote symptoms of each remedy are encircled. These keynotes are themes, such as "sore pains" or "burning pains" or "fear". These symptoms should be expected to appear no matter whether you are considering labor, hemorrhage, or after-pain symptoms. If a remedy such as Arsenicum is known for "burning pains", don't consider it for soreness. Or, if "fear" is a keynote, it's important to see that symptom in the total picture. Keynote symptoms are underlined in the text. PART 1 - Quick Reference Guide, has all of the encircled keynotes together for easy reference. Select your possibilities, read about them in greater detail in the text, and then, if possible, read in even greater detail in Kent's *Materia Medica* or in Yingling's *The Accoucheur's Emergency Manual.*

Remedies are also divided into "Warm" and "Chilly" remedies in PART 2 and PART 3. Most remedy pictures include the subjective experience of the patient ("I am cold" or "I feel hot") and so this was an attempt at helping the user to identify which grouping to consider. With some remedies however, hot and cold are not the determining symptoms; with many it is, and overall it made more sense to stay with this format. If chilly is listed in the keynote circle, then assume it <u>must</u> be a chilly remedy type (ie, the patient must be generally chilly for it to fit the picture and work effectively).

PART 4 - "The Baby" is meant for quick access if the child is in distress. Changes should be seen in seconds to one minute, especially if the baby is blue or listless. The more serious the symptom, the faster the response. If no change is seen, go onto the next remedy, or higher potency if you are convinced of your prescription.

This work is meant to be a stepping stone to the works referred to in the bibliography. It is always best to explore these remedies in greater detail when prescribing — especially if time permits.

Potency: For beginners the 30C potency is recommended. However, in birthing situations a higher potency like 200C or 1M may be required. Use your disgression; especially for the "baby-in-distress" remedies, a 200C may be preferable. Remedies in 30C may be repeated every 15-30 minutes in non-emergency conditions such as stimulating labor. In active hemorrhage or other emergencies you can repeat a 30C every few minutes. Improvement should be seen rapidly. If no change occurs, stop. A definitive change should be seen after one dose of a 200C, even if it needs to be repeated later.

<u>LEGEND</u>

> = better from
< = worse from
SXS = symptoms

I hope that the information presented here will open up a new world of homeopathy for you.

Jana Shiloh, M.A.

PART - 1

QUICK REFRENCE GUIDE

Chilly Remedy Type Keynotes

ARNICA - p.12

Face Hot, Flushed; Body Cool   Pains; Severe
PAINS: SORE, BRUISED   FATIGUE
Overly Ssensitive   Ailments from Injury

ARSENICUM ALBUM - p.13

Restless or Prostrate   Wants Company
Thirsty for small sips   **FEARFUL**   Burning pains > Heat
< 12-3 A.M   Chilly   Pale

BRYONIA - p.14

Irritable   < Noise   Thirsty for Cold
<Sitting Up   **SXS < ANY MOVEMENT**   Face Red, Hot
Wants to be Alone   Pains; Burning, Lancinating

CALCAREA CARBONICUM - p.15

Forehead Perspiration   Head Perspiration
Varicosities   **RESPONSIBLE**   Fair, Fat, Flabby
Craves Dairy - Eggs   Chilly   Can Crave Clay and Earth

CANTHARIS - p.16

Restlessness   Cutting Pains
Delirium   **BURNING PAINS IN BLADDER**   Anxiety
Prostration   Hypersensitivity

CARBO VEGETABILIS - p.17

No Restlessness   Gas   Pale or Bluish Skin
COLD BUT WANTS TO BE FANNED
Faint-like Weakness   Collapsed   Hot Head, Cold Body

CAULOPHYLLUM - p.18

Intermittent Pains   Nervous   Spasmodic Pains
FALSE, OR NON-PRODUCTIVE LABOR PAINS
Weakness   Irritable   Uterine debility

CHINA - p.19

Aversion to Being Touched   > Cool air
AILMENTS FROM FLUID LOSS (HEMORRHAGE)
Cold Sweat   Faint Pulse   Distention

CICUTA - p.20

SPASMS AND CONVULSIONS
< Touch and Noise

CIMICIFUGA - p.21

Rigors   Pains Fly From Side to Side   Pale or Bluish
Overly-Sensitive   **FEARFUL—POSSIBLY DERANGED**   Rheumatic Types
Pains; Sore, Bruised   Electric Shock-like Pains   Spasms, Cramps

COFFEA - p.22

Nervousness   Cannot Bear any Pain   Insomnia with Joy
OVERLY EXCITED, SENSITIVE AND IRRITABLE
<Touch   Fear of Death   Complaining   < Noise

GELSEMIUM - p.23

Bruised Feeling Throughout Body (See Arnica)
Frightened   **APATHETIC, DULL, WEAK**   Irritable
Trembling Weakness   Pains Run Upward

GOSSYPIUM. - p.24

RETAINED PLACENTA

HAMAMELIS - p.25

Does Not Feel Respected
HEMMORHOIDS AND VARICOSE VEINS
Burning Pains   Hemorrhage

HYPERICUM - p.26

INJURY TO THE NERVES & COCCYX
Lacerations

IGNATIA - p.27

Sighs Often   Hysterical Types   Restless
AILMENTS FROM GRIEF
Oversensitive to Pain   Consolation Irritates

IPECAC - p.28

Can be Chilly or Warm   Suffocative Breathing
CONSTANT NAUSEA
Pains From Left to Right of Abdomen   Cutting, Pinching Pains

KALI CARBONICUM - p.29

Restless   Shooting pains
Irritable   **BACK PAIN INTO BUTTOCKS, LEGS**   Thirst
Gas > burping   < Open Air

KREOSOTUM - p.30

Weakness Numbness Depressed
Irritable **OFFENSIVE, BURNING DISCHARGES** Tearful
Sharp Pains, or Bearing Down Burning Pains

LAC CANNINUM - p.31

Restless Depressed Milk-related
Can Curse **PAINS & SXS ALTERNATE SIDES** Feet Burn
Bearing Down Pains Sharp Darting Pains

LAUROCERASUS - p.32

Pale or Blue With Hemorrhage
GASPING FOR BREATH
Asphyxia in Baby Twitching of Muscles

MAGNESIUM PHOSPHORICUM - p.33

Excessive Expulsive Efforts < Cold Air Pains From Navel Outward
PAINS > HEAT AND PRESSURE
Leg Cramps in Labor Changing Pains Suffers Greatly

NUX MOSCHATA - p.34

SPACEY, SLEEPY
Confusion as if Intoxicated

NUX VOMICA - p.35

Irritable < Drafts or Cool Air < Touching
INEFFECTUAL URGING
Back Labor Chilly > Covering <3-5 AM

PHOSPHORUS - p.36

Wants People Near   Bruises and/or Bleeds Easily   Burning Pains
Fearful   **SYMPATHETIC, IMPRESSIONABLE**   Weakness
May Vomit as Cold Drink Warms in Stomach   Thirst for Very Cold Drinks
< Constipation: Stool Long, Narrow   <Noise, Odors, Lights

PLATINA - p.37

Great Sexual Escitement   Pain: Cramping
HIGH SEXUAL DESIRE or HAUGHTY & ARROGANT
Estreme Sensitivity of Genitals   Pain, as of a Vise or Tourniquet

RUTA - p.38

Sore All Over
PROLAPSED RECTUM AFTER DELIVERY
Miscarriages at 7 Months

SABINA - p.39

3 Month Miscarriages
PAINS FROM SACRUM TO PUBES
Weakness   Nervousness

SECALE - p.40

Bearing Down Pains   Black, Offensive Discharges   >Fresh Air or Fanning
COLD BUT < COVERING UP
Thin Women with Many Births   Burning Like Little Sparks on Body

SEPIA - p.41

All Gone Empty Feeling In Stomach   Flushes of Heat
Darting Pains Up from Cervix   **CHILLY**   Bearing Down Uterine Pains
Irritable   Weight in Anus as from Ball

QUICK REFERENCE GUIDE

Warm Remedy Type Keynotes

ACONITE - p.44

Restlessness	Predicts Hour of Death	Thirst
Dry Heat	**FEAR, TERROR**	Vertigo
Violent Pains	Flushed Face + Heat	Palpitations

APIS - p.45

Irritable   Piercing Shrieks
HOT STINGING PAINS
Heat   < Touch or Pressure   Thirstless

BELLADONNA - p.46

Pains, Sxs, Start and Stop Suddenly
Pupils Dilated, Red   **HOT, RED, VIOLENT**   < Noise, Light, Jarring Bed
Fearful   Throbbing Pains and Circulation   Moaning

CHAMOMILE - p.47

Cheeks Red or One Red, One Pale
< Company   **IRRITABLE, NASTY, FROM PAIN**   Thirst
Snappish, Rude, even Violent   Nothing Satisfies

LACHESIS - p.48

Cyanosis
< Constrictive Clothing   < Touching the Neck
SENSE OF CONSTRICTION
Women Near Menopause   Bearing Down Pains

LYCOPODIUM - p.49

Gas   Flushes of Facial Heat   Dry Vagina
RIGHT-SIDED PAINS, OR RIGHT TO LEFT
< 4-8 P.M.   Must Move with Pain   > Open Air

NATRUM MURIATICUM - p.50

Sad   Slow labor
< CONSOLATION, WANTS TO BE ALONE
Ailments from Grief   Craves Salt, Sour

PULSATILLA - p.51

Changeable symptoms   > Company and Consolation
SWEET and TEARFUL, OR TOUCHY and IRRITABLE
Slow Labor   Warm   > Open Air   >Slow walking
Often Blondes with Blue Eyes

PYROGENUM - p.52

Restless   **SEPTIC FEVERS**   Low Fever+ Rapid pulse
Discharges smell rotten

RUTA - p.53

Sore All Over
PROLAPSED RECTUM AFTER DELIVERY
Miscarriages at 7 Months

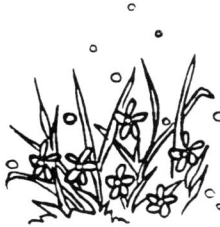

The following are some cases from my experience which may give you a sense of how a case may present:

I arrived to find the woman very fearful, her eyes were round with fear, and her pupils were contracted. She was breathing heavily. When questioned, she admitted she felt that she would die that night. She was afraid to continue with the labor, and shrieked with each contraction. The remedy relaxed her, the fear melted, and labor progressed.

She was whimpering and tearful, feeling she just could not go on any longer. All the windows were open, and she wanted to be near the windows or to be outside. She was holding onto her husband, wanting his reassurances, which helped only temporarily and then she would become despondant again. When the midwife tried to be firm with her she wailed "don't rush me", and broke down into tears. Pains became slow and irregular. She refused to drink much water. One dose of a 1m changed the nature of the contractions and gave this woman the inner strength to complete the delivery.

Back pains were severe and she cried for pressure on her sacrum with each contraction. The pains radiated into the buttocks. After the correct remedy the labor pains changed in one contraction.

She was warm, nasty and irritable, shrieking with each contraction. She ordered her helpers to do first one thing and then another but each time they complied she told them they weren't doing it right and changed her request. She had back labor but the pains extended down the inner thighs. For all of her pains, labor was unproductive. A few minutes after a 200c her whole demeanor changed and she delivered shortly thereafter.

Remedies given: #1:Aconite, #2: Pulsatilla, #3: Kali carbonicum #4: Chamomile

PART - 2

CHILLY REMEDIES TYPES

ARNICA

Face Hot, Flushed; Body Cool   Pains; Severe

PAINS: SORE, BRUISED / FATIGUE

Overly-sensitive   Ailments from injury

PREGNANCY: With bruised sore pains from foetal movement. Also sensation that the foetus is lying cross-wise.

LABOR: False labor pains when accompanied by a sense of soreness in one part, or throughout. Fatigue of uterus resulting in weak contractions. Severe unproductive pains. Great sense of soreness in body as though the bed were too hard; no position is comfortable. Sore pains in the back. Vaginal area too sensitive to be examined. Head hot, body cooler. Soreness of uterus with pressure of child's head. Dribbling of urine after labor. Can be used during labor, and after the birth routinely for trauma to the body from giving birth .

HEMORRHAGE: From injury, fatigue, shock. Bright red flow with or without clots, and a sense of soreness. Pain may or may not be present. Nausea. After long labor, trauma, instrument delivery.

MISCARRIAGE: Threatened or real, from injury (also Rhus Tox), concussion, or shock. Bright red blood. Pain on movement of mother, or child. Threatened septicemia after miscarriage or abortion.

AFTER PAINS: Can avert pains when given in a high potency after the birth if labor involved much bruising to parts. It will assist in returning uterus to normal shape, and will help protect against infection. For pains in uterus with nursing.

THE BABY: For any bruising or injury during or at the time of birth. Instrument deliveries. **Asphyxia.** Face hot, body cold; face hot, nose cold, jerking breath; tremor in limbs.

ARSENICUM ALBUM

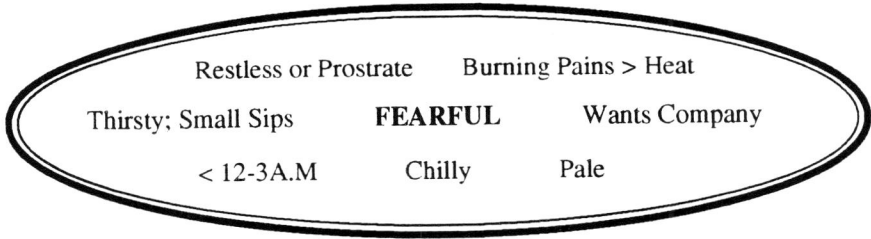

Restless or Prostrate   Burning Pains > Heat

Thirsty; Small Sips   **FEARFUL**   Wants Company

< 12-3A.M   Chilly   Pale

PREGNANCY: Heart burn when foetus lodges against pyloric valve. All keynote symptoms apply. So fearful wants to go to hospital, or have midwife around, before due date.

LABOR: Exhaustion after every effort (prostration). Rigid vagina: will hardly admit a finger. Urine retention after labor (also Causticum). Fearful, will not be left alone. Fears death.

HEMORRHAGE: Dark. Burning and lancinating pains.

BABY: Tetanic spasms. Lies pale, warm, but as if dead. Breathless, distorted features. Stiff knees and feet. Dry skin.

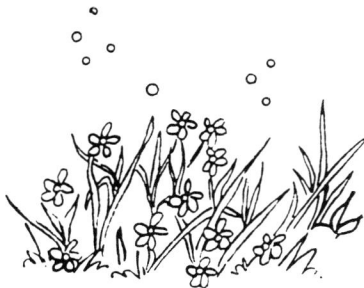

BRYONIA

Irritable   < Noise   Thirsty for Cold

<Sitting Up   **SXS < ANY MOVEMENT**   Face Red, Hot

Wants to be Alone   Pains;' Burning, Lancinating

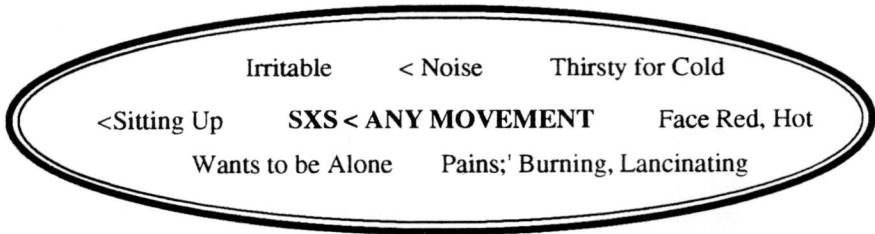

This remedy chills easily but feels hot internally.

PREGNANCY: Nausea < motion.

LABOR: Pains < any movement. Sighing (see Ignatia). Drawing or lancinating pains from hip to foot.

HEMORRHAGE: Bleeding occurs with slightest motion, even on deep inhalation or movement of foot. Dark red blood with headache. Often seen in Brunettes

MISCARRIAGE: Dark red blood, dry constipated stool. Pains throughout body, <motion. Headache <motion.

AFTER-PAINS: <motion of any kind, even on deep breathing.

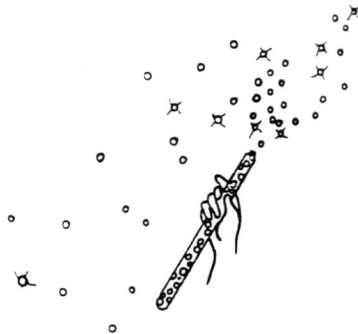

CALCAREA CARBONICUM

Forehead Perspiration   Head Perspiration

Varicosities   **RESPONSIBLE**   Fair, Fat, Flabby

Craves dairy -Eggs   Chilly   Can Crave Clay and Earth

Indications for this remedy lie in the general constitutional picture presented in abbreviated keynote form here. Reference Yingling and Kent's lectures on the Materia Medica for further confirmatory information.

PREGNANCY: If other keynote symptoms apply: Varices of sexual organs, legs and leg cramps.

HEMORRHAGE: Profuse bright red blood. Painless.

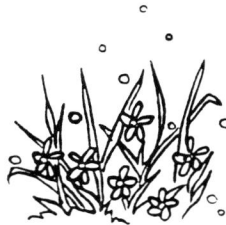

Chilly Remedy Types

15

CANTHARIS

Delirium   Restlessness   Anxiety

BURNING PAINS IN BLADDER

Cutting Pains   Hypersensitivity   Prostration

During any condition of miscarriage, labor, hemorrhage, or retained placenta, there will be a constant urging to urinate, passing only a few drops of urine (or none), with violent cutting and/or burning pains. (See Nux Vomica)

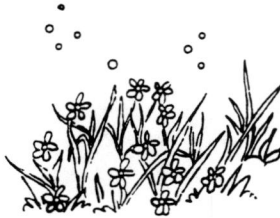

CARBO VEGETABILIS

No Restlessness   Gas   Pale or Bluish Skin

COLD BUT WANTS TO BE FANNED

Faint-like Weakness   Collapsed   Hot Head, Cold Body

PREGNANCY: All keynotes apply. May include difficult respiration because of fullness in abdomen. Some forms of asthma during pregnany in those who never had problems before; keynotes apply for asthma symtoms too.

LABOR: Too weak, or pains stop from weakness. Varicose veins of vulva. Weakness from debilitating disease, or loss of fluid (also see China). Much belching.

MISCARRIAGE: with varicosity of sexual organs, frequent headache, abdominal spasms.

HEMORRHAGE: Passive, continuous, near collapse, bluish or deathly pale skin. Pulse rapid and weak, chilly, wanting to be fanned. Cold sweat, as if dead. No anxiety. Difficulty breathing, burning pains-chest, sacrum.

AFTER-PAINS: In other parts of pelvis, not uterus.

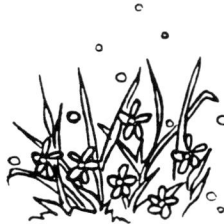

CAULOPHYLLUM

Intermittent Pains   Nervous   Spasmodic Pains

FALSE, OR NON-PRODUCTIVE LABOR PAINS

Weakness   Uterine debility   Irritable

LABOR: False labor pains. Short, intermittent labor pains that are non-productive. Pains fly all over. Os: rigid, pain like needles in cervix. Pains slow from exhaustion, but spasms severe. Severe pains in early labor. Much vaginal mucus. Nausea.

MISCARRIAGE: Very minimal bleeding, emphasis on pain. Lack of uterine tonicity. From hysteria, uterine inertia, or congestion. Also in rheumatic patients.

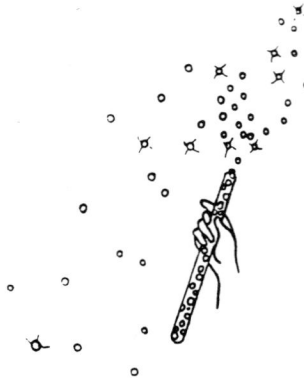

CHINA

Aversion to Being Touched   > Cool Air

AILMENTS FROM LOSS OF FLUIDS (HEMORRHAGE)

Cold Sweat   Faint Pulse   Distention

LABOR: Pains stop with hemorrhage. Skin so sensitive does not want to be touched; light touch is painful. Exhaustion from loss of fluids. Cold skin, ringing in ears. Nervous. Vertigo. Distention of gas without relief. Highly sensitive nervous system, < noise, touch, excitement. Hot face, cold body.

MISCARRIAGE: Sense of bloated abdomen. Constant hemorrhage with weakness, pallor, almost pulseless, and limp. All kinds of discharge.

HEMORRHAGE AND RETAINED PLACENTA: Atony of uterus. With much loss of blood; heaviness of head, vertigo, ringing in ears, fainting, vanishing of senses, gasping for breath, cold, pale, blue face and hands, and delusions on closing eyes. Wants to be fanned.

CONVULSIONS: From great loss of blood. Throbbing carotids, flushed (See Belladonna, Aconite).

THE BABY: Lifeless (syncope) as a result of great blood loss by mother during labor.

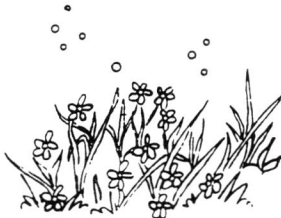

CICUTA

LABOR: Violent contortions and spasms of head, face and body during or after labor. Spasms < touch, noise. Trembling of left leg.

THE BABY: Spasmodic rigidity, with frequent jerking.

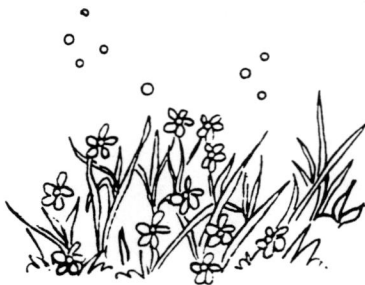

CIMICIFUGA

Rigors   Pains Fly From Side to Side   Pale or Bluish

Overly-Sensitive   **FEARFUL**   Rheumatic Types
Pains; Sore, Bruised   **POSSIBLY DERANGED**   Spasms, Cramps

Electric Shock-like Pains

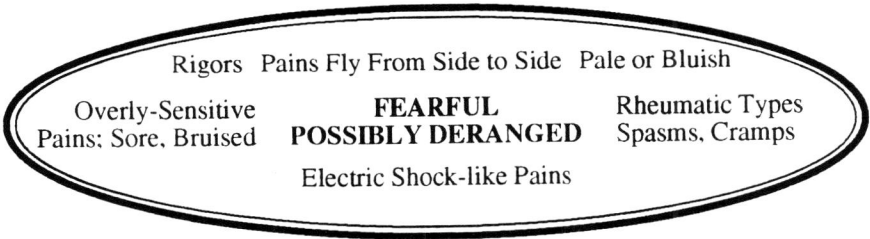

PREGNANCY: This remedy has been given by some doctors once per week during the month before delivery.

LABOR: False labor pains even weeks early. Rigors and chills in early labor (see Gels). Pains fly from one side to the other of abdomen (also see Ipecac, left to right; and Lycopodium, right to left), not in uterus. Irregular dilation; dilated, then closed shut. Irregular constriction of os, often with bleeding. Cramping in hips. Fearful and nervous, a sense of foreboding that something bad is going to happen (see Arsenicum). Depressed, may fear insanity, or be suspicious. May cry out in agony. Nonsensical talk. Changes subject often, fears death. Twitching, trembling of legs. Pain in heart extending down left arm.

MISCARRIAGE: At 3 months. Pains fly from side to side of abdomen. Recurrent miscarriages in women who have rheumatic problems. Pain in back, extending down legs.

HEMORRHAGE: Labor-like pains, ceasing with flow. Passive, dark, coagulated. Pains in back, extending into limbs.

RETAINED PLACENTA: Severe tearing pains, uterine inactivity. Headache, brain feels like it will burst. Rheumatic patients.

AFTER-PAINS: Cannot tolerate pain; overly-sensitive. Pains focused in groins. Tenderness in uterus < pressure. Flushing of face. Depressed, restless, sleepless.

COFFEA

Nervousness   Cannot Bear Any Pain   Insomnia with Joy

OVERLY-EXCITED, SENSITIVE and IRRITABLE

Fear of Death   < Noise   Complaining   <Touch

This remedy looks similar to Cimicifuga, but some of the specifics are different. For example, the headache: it feels contracted, not bursting. Note other differences as you read the specifics.

LABOR: Back labor. Her great sensitivity causes crying, whining and fear of death. Loquacious. False labor pains with facial neuralgia. Labor pains may cease. May predict hour of death (see Aconite) Rigidity of vulva and perineum. Nervous excitement. Can faint with fear.

MISCARRIAGE: From too much excitement. Extremely severe pains.

HEMORRHAGE: Large black lumps < each motion. Violent pains in groin. Sexual organs sensitive to any touch (see Arnica, Platina). Itching, but she dares not scratch due to sensitivity.

AFTER-PAINS: Extremely painful not consistent to contractions. Fears death. Cannot sleep due to over-excitement.

GELSEMIUM

Bruised Feeling Throughout Body (see Arnica)

Frightened   **APATHETIC, DULL, WEAK**   Irritable

Trembling Weakness   Pains Run Upward.

PREGNANCY: Anxiety before labor. Can be given in advance of labor when fear is present.

LABOR: Os hard, thick, rigid and undilatable. False labor pains. Chills and rigors. Uterine inertia. Pains cease while os is widely dilated. Pains change, run up back and to hips. She can be drowsy and flushed or fearful and nervous. Muscles weak, trembling (especially legs). Tongue trembles when extended out. Looks dazed and dull. Face flushed, dark red, or pale or sickly. Other pains interrupt labor. Baby seems to ascend with each pain. Nervous trembling and chattering during and after labor. Intermittent pulse. Fearful anticipation and hysteria (see Coffea).

MISCARRIAGE, AND AFTER-PAINS: Sharp Pains run upward and up back. Chills up back. Lack of strong muscular control; weakness, trembling. Ailments from fright (see Aconite) and fear of events to come.

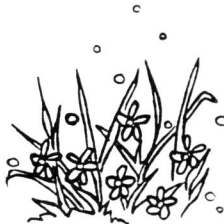

GOSSYPIUM

RETAINED PLACENTA

No generalities but some useful specifics.

LABOR: Feeble contractions, nearly painless.

MISCARRIAGE: Foetus is expelled <u>leaving placenta in place</u>, with closed os.

RETAINED PLACENTA: Often after premature delivery. <u>Placenta will not loosen no matter what is done</u>.

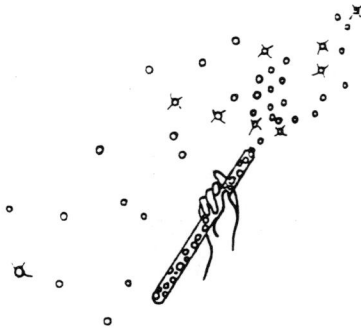

HAMAMELIS

Does not feel respected

HEMMORHOIDS AND VARICOSE VEINS

Burning pains   Hemorrhage

Not many general symptoms, but known for knotty, painful varicose veins, and hemorrhoids, and also one of several possibilities for varicosities of the genitalia (see Calcarea Carb, Carbo Veg and Lycopodium)

HEMORRHAGE: Is < by day, stops at night. Slow, steady and passive; bright red, or dark.

MISCARRIAGE: Sore abdomen, continuous red bleeding.

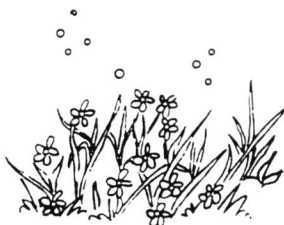

HYPERICUM

INJURY TO NERVES AND COCCYX

Lacerations

This first aid remedy is for injury to the nerves. It should be used if there is <u>injury to the coccyx</u> in childbirth or pain in labor, or <u>for tearing during childbirth</u> (not for episiotomy - use Staphyagria).

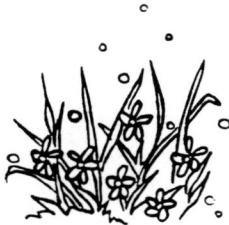

IGNATIA

Sighs Often   Hysterical Types   Restless

AILMENTS FROM GRIEF

Oversensitive to Pain   Consolation Irritates

PREGNANCY: Fear of losing the child (especially when she had a hard time conceiving).

LABOR: Pains feeble or stopping. Rigid os. Legs tremble. Crying. Usually occurring when a painful experience is affecting the woman, such as a recent death or heartbreak. In such cases, give one dose prior to labor in a 200C or 1M potency.

MISCARRIAGE, HEMORRHAGE, AND AFTER-PAINS: Sinking empty feeling in uterus or stomach. Ailments from grief, obvious or suppressed. Much sadness with sighing.

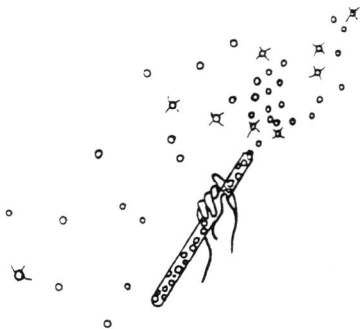

IPECAC

PREGNANCY: <u>Constant nausea</u>, not amelorated by vomiting. Tongue remains clean and uncoated.

LABOR: Cutting, pinching pain near navel shoots to uterus interrupting contraction. Pains cut across abdomen left to right. <u>Nausea with clean tongue</u>.

MISCARRIAGE: Continuous, steady flow of bright red blood, so severe it may flow over the foot of the bed. <u>Nausea</u> and clots. Cutting pains in abdomen, left to right.

HEMORRHAGE AND RETAINED PLACENTA: <u>With or without nausea</u>. Continuous, steady, profuse. Cold, shuddering. Cold sweat. Dizzy, pale, gasping. Gushes at each effort to vomit.

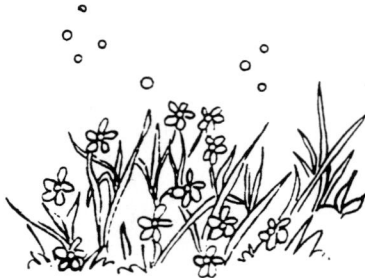

KALI CARBONICUM

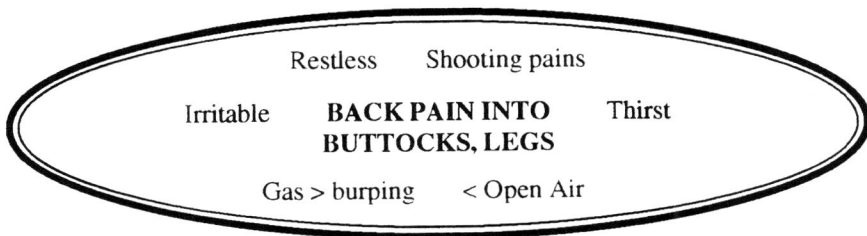

Restless   Shooting pains

Irritable   **BACK PAIN INTO**   Thirst
BUTTOCKS, LEGS

Gas > burping   < Open Air

LABOR: <u>Back labor</u>. Sharp, cutting pains in lumbar stopping labor, extending into buttocks and legs. > pressure. Pulsation in arteries. < open air, weeps much. Swelling above eyelids. Hour-glass contractions. Pains cease or are too weak.

MISCARRIAGE: At 2-3 months. <u>Lumbar pains < walking, > sitting</u> or lying. Swelling over eyes.

HEMORRHAGE: <u>Sharp pains from lumbar to buttocks</u>. A major remedy for post-partum hemorrhage.

AFTER-PAINS: <u>Lumbar into gluteal region, or hips</u>. May extend downward.

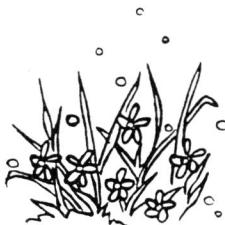

KREOSOTUM

Weakness   Numbness   Depressed

Irritable   **OFFENSIVE, BURNING DISCHARGES**   Burning Pains

Sharp Pains, or Bearing Down   Tearful

PREGNANCY: Great salivation during pregnancy. Feels she vomits because of salivation (see Mercurius also for salivation, especially during sleep). <u>Vaginitis with severe burning</u> < after urination, < walking. Bleeds after coition.

MISCARRIAGE: At 3rd month. Dark offensive discharges, intermittent, watery, lumpy.

HEMORRHAGE: < lying down, ceases on standing. Dark blood, is acrid, irritating the body. May stop and resume later. <u>Bearing down pains</u>.

LAC CANNINUM

Restless   Depressed   Milk-related

Cursing   **PAINS & SXS, ALTERNATE SIDES**   Feet Burn

Bearing Down Pains   Sharp Darting Pains

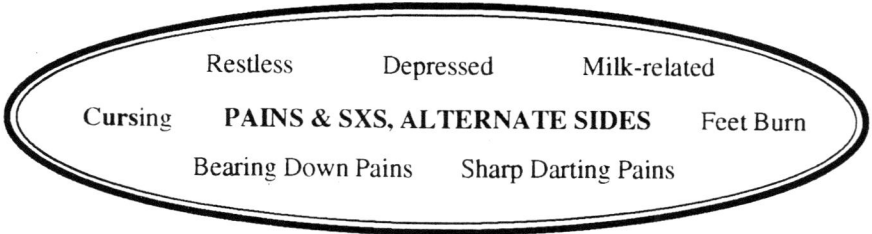

LABOR: Sharp pains extending upwards in uterus. Severely retroverted uterus. Swelling of left labia.

HEMORRHAGE: Blood hot as fire. Stringy, clotting. Bearing down pains as if everything would fall out. <u>Ovarian pains alternate sides</u>.

AFTER-PAINS: Severe pains shooting down legs, < right side.

BREASTS: For caked knotty breasts after miscarriage. Dries up milk.

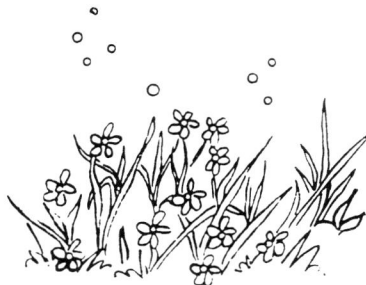

LAUROCERASUS

Pale or Blue With Hemorrhage

GASPING FOR BREATH

Asphyxia in Baby   Twitching of Muscles

PREGNANCY: Gastritis during pregnancy, > lying on back. Palpitations may occur with gastritis. Aversion to food.

HEMORRHAGE: Cold, pale, clammy, from loss of blood. Dimness of vision. Gasping of breath.

THE BABY: Asphyxia. Blue Face, gasping for breath or imperceptible breathing. Twitching in face.

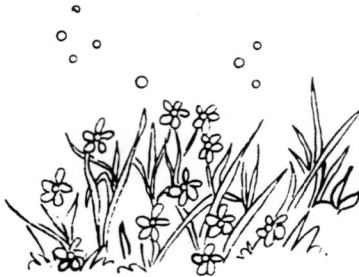

MAGNESIUM PHOSPHORICUM

Excessive Expulsive Efforts   Pains From Navel Outward

< Cold Air   **PAINS > HEAT AND PRESSURE**   Suffers Greatly

Leg Cramps in Labor   Changing Pains

There's not much more to report here, it's all above.

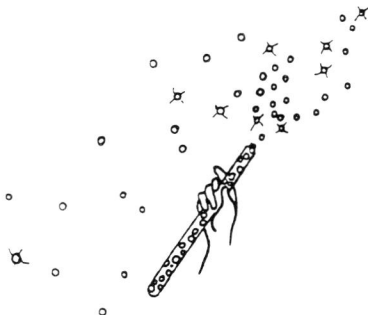

NUX MOSCHATA

SPACEY, SLEEPY
Confusion as if Iintoxicated

PREGNANCY: Spacey and difficult to think. Menses may come during first three months of pregnancy.

LABOR: Sleepy before and during labor. (also see Gelsemium and Opium which is mentioned in Yingling, but is no longer sold in the U.S.)

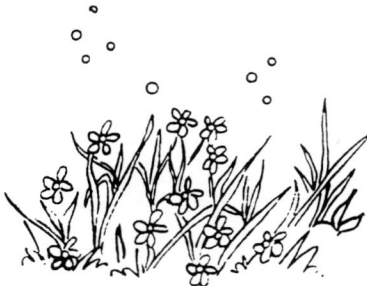

NUX VOMICA

Irritable   < Drafts or Cool Air   < Touching

INEFFECTUAL URGING

Back Labor   Chilly > Covering   <3-5 A.M.

Generally seen in high-strung women who are very stressed and nervous, and crave stimulants. Also in those with a sedentary lifestyle. The theme of ineffectual urging is best put as "wants to, but can't" whether that be for stool, vomiting, or urinating.

PREGNANCY: Sensitive to odors, much retching, but may have difficulty vomiting.

LABOR: Pains so intense they stop dilation. Back labor extending to buttocks and thighs (like Kali carb. but the Nux v. pain is < with pressure). Pains accompanied with constant urgings for stool, with no bowel movement. Irritable, can be abusive.

MISCARRIAGES: From stimulants or drugs or toxins.

HEMORRHAGES: Accompanied with large difficult stools, or frequent urging with little or no results. Bright red lumpy clots.

AFTER-PAINS: Violent and protracted; aching and sore. She does not want to be disturbed, irritable. Desire for stool with each pain.

PHOSPHORUS

> Fearful   Bruises and/or Bleeds Easily   Weakness
> Wants People Near **SYMPATHETIC, IMPRESSIONABLE** Burning Pains
> Thirst for Very Cold Drinks   Constipation: Stool Long, Narrow
> <Noise, Odors, Lights   May Vomit as Cold Drink Warms in Stomach.

Tall, thin, delicate women with reddish hair are more likely to need Phosphorus.

PREGNANCY: <u>Anxiety for others</u>. Nausea with sense of emptiness. Skin bruises easily. She may feel "spacey".

LABOR: Non-productive painful contractions. Sense of weakness in abdomen. <u>Copious bleeding, bright red</u>. <u>Craves ice cold drinks</u>, sodas, sweets, ice cream and salt.

MISCARRIAGE: Uterine weakness. <u>Burning</u>, throbbing pain on top of head and forehead. Nausea and vomiting < A.M. to noon. <u>Profuse and continuous bleeding</u> of bright red blood.

HEMORRHAGE: Tall, thin women. <u>Copious bleeding</u> after difficult labor, may be intermittent. Abdomen:cold and weak, < touch. Sacral pains, < any motion. Flushes of heat upwards. <u>Also heavy bleeding in nursing women</u>.

PLATINA

Great sexual excitement   Pain: Cramping
HIGH SEXUAL DESIRE or HAUGHTY & ARROGANT
Extreme Sensitivity of Genitals   Pain, as of a Vise or Tourniquet

LABOR: <u>Extreme sensitivity vagina</u> and os, cannot stand to be touched. Inefficient pains, weak. Hour-glass contractions. Severe cramping. Oozing of dark blood. Left-sided labor pains. Cries with pain. After labor, <u>so sensitive cannot stand napkin against her</u>. Hysterical mania.

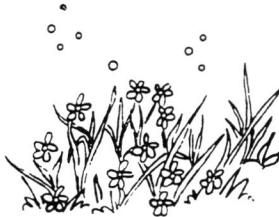

RUTA

Sore all over

PROLAPSED RECTUM AFTER DELIVERY

Miscarriages at 7 months

MISCARRIAGE: At seven months, resulting in a long and slow recovery.

SABINA

3 Month Miscarriages

PAINS FROM SACRUM TO PUBES

Weakness   Nervousness

LABOR: Pain from sacrum to pubes or vice versa. Flushes of heat in face with chilly body.

MISCARRIAGE: At around the 3rd month, pain as in labor. Hemorrhage predominates. Bright red blood with clots, followed by dark red blood with clots like pieces of liver. < every motion. Many different kinds of bleeding.

HEMORRHAGE: < Slightest motion but > walking around. Pain or discomfort, sacrum to pubes. Often with pain in joints, and weakness. Profuse, offensive, clotted. Liver-like clots.

RETAINED PLACENTA: Intense pains with retained placenta. Pains or uneasiness from sacrum to pubes. Fluid blood and clots in equal parts, with each pain.

SECALE

Bearing Down Pains
Black, Offensive Discharges   > Fresh Air or Fanning

COLD BUT < COVERING UP

Burning Like Little Sparks on Body
Thin Women with Many Births

LABOR: Cold skin with a cold sweat, but averse to covering up. Can feel a sense of a burning, *and* cold < covering, > cold air, or wants to be fanned. Seen in scrawny, thin, wrinkled women after many births. Pains cease or are non-productive. Any emotional state from apathy to great anguish. Pains in fingers; does not want them touching each other. Discharges black and offensive. Hour-glass contractions, Prolonged bearing down pains. Everything seems loose and open without action.

MISCARRIAGE: Third month, with copious black, offensive discharge, with black clots; or intermittent with red gushes. Discharge predominates, labor-like pains alternating with hemorrhage. Tingling all over. > fresh air or wants to be fanned.

HEMORRHAGE: Same symptoms as miscarriage, passive, < motion.

RETAINED PLACENTA: Constant, strong sensation of bearing down, yet ineffectual pains. Hour-glass contractions. Too relaxed for uterine action. Chilly but < warmth or covering.

AFTER PAINS: Elderly thin, scrawny, multiparae women, or after primiparae. Frequent, tonic, labor-like pains, thin, brown, offensive lochia. All other keynotes apply.

SEPIA

Flushes of Heat   All Gone Empty Feeling in Stomach

Irritable   **CHILLY**   BearingDown Uterine Pains

Darting Pains Up From Cervix   Weight in Anus as from Ball

PREGNANCY: Nausea < odor of foods. Sex drive low or non-existant, and aversion to husband. Very irritable and often depressed. < 3-5 P.M. Lumbar pain > lying on hard floor with book pressing into back. Herpetic eruptions if other symptoms agree.

LABOR: Induration of cervix and rigid uterus. Darting needle-like pain upwards. Weak pains. Shuddering. Flushes of heat. Empty feeling in stomach.

PREGNANCY or LABOR: Cold hands and feet. Sadness or indifference. Irritable and "touchy". Aversion to husband. Fearful, and fretful. < smell of food. Yellow or brown spots on face, or yellow saddle across nose. Uterus sore from activity of foetus. Palpitations with emotions. Hysterical spasms. Constipation. Violent aversion to smoke.

MISCARRIAGE: Tendency to abort in the 5th to 7th month. Sensation of weight in anus as from a ball. Flushes of heat with faintness. Labor-like pain in uterus.

HEMORRHAGES: Congestion with sense of weight. Pain in right groin, and/or needle-like pains in cervix. Desires to draw legs up. Feels bearing down pains as if everything would fall out of uterus. Cold with flushes of heat. Constipated. Putrid odor of urine.

RETAINED PLACENTA: Same symptoms as above. Consider Sepia and Pulsatilla where no symptoms are present after miscarriage.

AFTER PAINS: Mostly felt in back; bearing down and severe. Vaginal pains shooting upward from vagina. Weight in anus as of a ball. This is a major remedy for post-partem depression.

PART - 3

WARM REMEDY TYPES

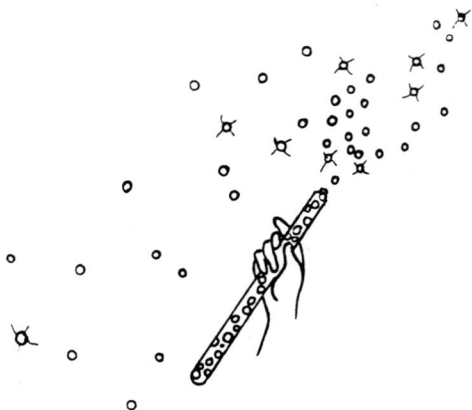

ACONITE

> Restlessness   Predicts Hour of Death   Thirst
>
> Dry Heat   **FEAR, TERROR**   Vertigo
>
> Violent Pains   Flushed Face + Heat   Palpitations

LABOR: The vulva, vagina and os are <u>dry</u>, tender, undilatable. <u>Restlessness</u>. Unproductive <u>violent</u> frequent pains cause <u>anxiety</u>. Sensitivity of vagina makes examination impossible. <u>Fears death, or impending doom</u>. <u>Usually dry heat</u>, but may have hot sweat.

MISCARRIAGE: <u>From fright</u> with anger or fear. From cystitis. Hemorrhage of bright red blood. More bleeding than pain. <u>Fears death</u>. <u>Vertigo</u> on rising.

HEMORRHAGE: <u>Fear of death</u>. Active bleeding. Fear of moving or turning over. <u>Dizzy</u> on sitting or standing up.

AFTER PAINS: <u>Fearful</u>. <u>Painful, strong</u>, last too long.

THE BABY: <u>Asphyxia</u>. <u>Hot, purplish</u> color, breathless, little or no perceptible pulse. Retained urine. Use when child has been traumatized, or even when crying after birth. Great for <u>birth trauma</u> of any sort.

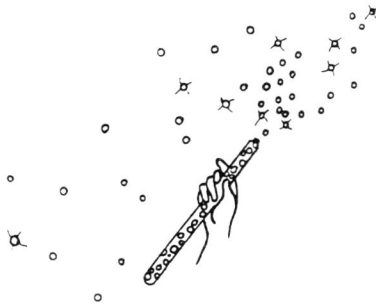

APIS

Irritable   Piercing Shrieks

HOT STINGING PAINS

Heat   < Touch or Pressure   Thirstless

This remedy comes from the bee. Think in terms of an angry bee and a sting.

PREGNANCY: Consider this remedy for albuminaria, but only if symptoms agree. Add to keynotes: hot with sense of suffocation. Dizziness < lying and closing eyes. Hysterical with strong irritability. Eyes, face, and/or ankles swollen in A.M. Hot flashes. Tearful.

MISCARRIAGE: In 2nd, 3rd and 4th months. Stinging pain in ovary(s) until labor-like pains occur, then extending into legs. Urine usually scanty. No thirst. Restless. Constipation. Yawning. Tearful. < Touch, light pressure. Sense of suffocation.

HEMORRHAGE: Active, dark, profuse. Restless. Yawning. Red spots (like bee stings) on skin. Stinging in ovaries. Symptoms may be brought on by hatred or jealousy. < Touch or light pressure. Tearful.

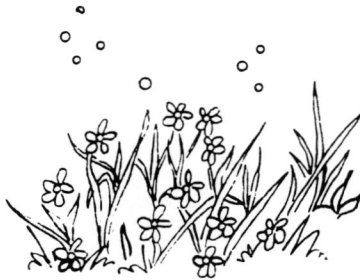

BELLADONNA

Pains, Sxs, Start and Stop Suddenly

Pupils Dilated, Red   **HOT, RED, VIOLENT** < Noise, Light, Jarring Bed

Fearful   Throbbing Pains and Circulation   Moaning

This remedy resembles Aconite, and in some cases, also Lachesis, so consider both as other options.

LABOR AND AFTER-PAINS: Suited to older women; primiparae. Labor stops and starts suddenly, violently, too quick bearing down. Os has spasmodic contractions, or hour-glass pains. Os rigid, thin, hot, red, more moist than Aconite. Labor slow, baby does not move. After water breaks, os spasmodically contracted. Pains may cease. Face flushed, hot, eyes may be glazed, bloodshot. Throbbing carotids. Moaning, may become delirious, even violent in nature.

MISCARRIAGE: Blood is hot. Pains and discharge stop and start suddenly. Back pain as if broken. All keynotes and labor information applies.

THE BABY: Red face, **Asphyxia**, dilated pupils, eyes staring, inability to swallow, spasmodic respiration.

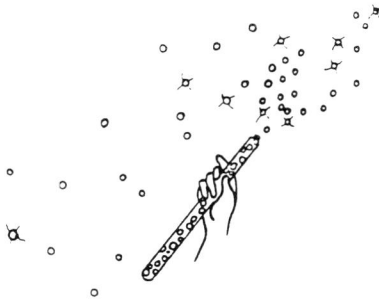

CHAMOMILE

Cheeks Red OR One Red, One Pale

< Company   **IRRITABLE, NASTY, FROM PAIN**   Thirst

Snappish, Rude, even Violent   Nothing Satisfies

LABOR AND RETAINED PLACENTA: Irritable to the extreme. Nasty. Cannot be satisfied. Pains - intolerable. Tearing pains in back extending down inner sides of legs. Blood discharged dark, coagulated, or clots. Hour-glass contractions. Needs fresh air. Pains non-productive. Rigid os. Large clots pass. One cheek may be pale, one red. Pains cause child to ascend. Restless. Irritable. She is intolerant of the slightest pain.

HEMORRHAGE: Dark, coagulated + red gushes. Irregular flow. Violent pains. Ailments from anger. Flushed, or one cheek pale, one red. Uterus in small knots. Copious, colorless, urine.

AFTER-PAINS: Severe irritability with severe pain. All keynote symptoms apply.

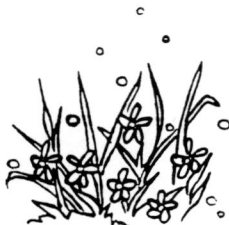

LACHESIS

Cyanosis

< Constrictive Clothing   < Touching the Neck

< SENSE OF CONSTRICTION

Women Near Menopause   Bearing Down Pains

PREGNANCY: Hair falls out. Right sided sciatica. Intolerance of rings, wristwatches and turtlenecks.

LABOR: Generally left-sided symptoms, except can be right when ovary is involved. Contracted os, with throat or heart symptoms. Women near climacteric. Emotionally can be angry, explosive, jealous, sad, or gloomy. Constipation, anus feels closed. < touch especially around throat. Flushes of heat. < After sleep: wakes into full blown symptoms. Loquacious, suspicious, < company.

HEMORRHAGE: Severe pain right ovary extending to uterus which increases until relieved by gush of blood.

THE BABY: Cyanosis (blue in face, nails, extremities)

LYCOPODIUM

Gas   Flushes of Facial Heat   Dry Vagina

RIGHT-SIDED PAINS, OR RIGHT TO LEFT

< 4-8 P.M.   Must Move with Pain   > Open Air

PREGNANCY: Gas with sense of distension. Weakness and faintness with hunger. Appetite either voracious, or she can fill easily with only a few bites of food. Irritable. some or all symptoms ≤ 4-8 P.M. Energy or symptoms then improve after 8 P.M.

LABOR: Pains move upward, OR right to left. Patient must move with the pain. Os spasmodic, undilated. Pains too weak; ceasing. Retention of urine due to severe pressure during labor (also see Causticum). Red sand in urine. Sense as if she would die from weakness. Gas, distention. Symptoms are worse 4-8 P.M.

MISCARRIAGE: Tendency for miscarriage. Severe pain in lumbar-sacral area, < before urination, > during flow. Dryness in vagina. Pains move from right to left.

HEMORRHAGE: Profuse, prolonged, part black clots, part red, part serum. < with stool.

AFTER PAINS: With sticking pains in right or left illiac region. Urging but unable to urinate. Bearing down pains.

NATRUM MURIATICUM

Sad Slow labor

< CONSOLATION, WANTS TO BE ALONE

Ailments from Grief Craves Salt, Sour, Fish

More of a constitutional remedy, but these keynotes will clue you into the type. It would help to read more about this remedy in Kent's "Materia Medica".

PREGNANCY: Sadness during pregnancy, often over a rejection, but <u>aversion to being consoled</u>. Cannot cry easily, especially in front of others. Herpes, if other sxs agree. Vertigo. Chilly *or* warm.

LABOR: Slow labor with feeble pains. Prolapsed uterus. Throbbing headache, < 10 am to 3 pm. A sadness with a sense of doom. May <u>pull away when affection is</u> given.

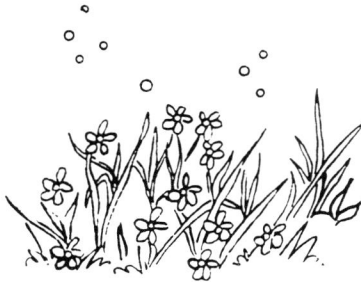

PULSATILLA

Changeable symptoms   > Company and Consolation
SWEET and TEARFUL, OR TOUCHY and IRRITABLE
Slow Labor   Warm   > Open Air   >Slow walking
Often Blondes with Blue Eyes

PREGNANCY: All keynotes apply. If other symptoms agree, consider for recurrent cystitis during pregnancy, varicose veins and/or involuntary urination with coughing and sneezing.

LABOR: Symptoms and moods are changeable. Patient will elicit your sympathy. Pains slow or ceasing. Uterine inertia. Hour glass contractions. Needs open air, room feels stuffy. Wants to move gently, like slow walking or motion to relieve pain. Pains on left forcing her to double over. Cutting pains, with sense of urging to stool (like Nux. vom). Back labor. *Will often right abnormal presentations* when used in a 200C or 1M, and when symptoms agree; not useful after the water breaks. Tearful and changeable mood > consolation. Thirstless. Impressionable and easily convinced or reassured. May be sleepy before and during labor. Affectionate; wants to be held or carressed.

MISCARRIAGE: Black or changeable blood. Stops and starts with renewed violence. Pains alternate with bleeding. < warm, stuffy room. Tearful, changeable mood > consolation, company.

AFTER-PAINS AND HEMORRHAGES: < Evening, < warm room, > consolation and reassurance,

PLACENTA: Inertia of uterus. Redness and soreness of hypogastrium. < touch. Retention of urine. Tearful and "mild" women (often blondes).

PYROGENUM

Restless   **SEPTIC FEVERS**   Low Fever+ Rapid pulse
Discharges Smell Rotten

MISCARRIAGE AND HEMORRHAGE: Bright red with clots.
Septic disease. Close to Ipecac, try one if the other fails.

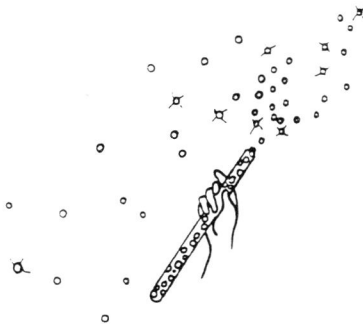

RUTA

Sore All Over

PROLAPSED RECTUM AFTER DELIVERY

Miscarriages at 7 Months

(Also listed under Part 2 - Chilly Remedy Types)

MISCARRIAGE: At seven months resulting in a long and slow recovery.

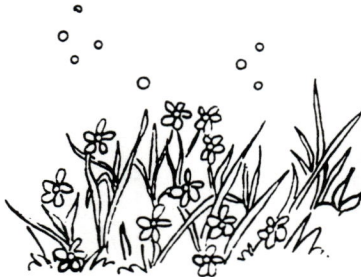

PART - 4

THE BABY

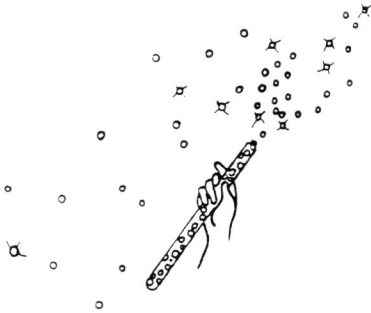

ACONITE: Asphyxia (also consider Arnica, Belladonna, Antimonium tart, and Laurocerasus). Hot, can have a **purplish** color, may be breathless with little or no perceptible pulse. Retained urine. Use when child has been traumatized, or even when crying after birth. Great for **birth trauma** of any sort. Also use for retention of urine after birth. Jaundice. For bad effects on infant's eyes from oxygen.

ARNICA: For any bruising or **injury** during or at the time of birth. Instrument deliveries. **Asphyxia. Face hot, body cold;** jerking breath; tremor in limbs. Also for hematomas.

ARSENICUM: Tetanic spasms. Lies pale, warm, but lifeless. **Breathless,** distorted features. Stiff knees and feet. Dry skin.

ANTIMONIUM TART: for **rattling** in throat or lungs of newborns. Face may be pale.

BELLADONNA: Red, hot face, Asphyxia dilated pupils, eyes staring, inability to swallow, spasmodic respiration.

CHINA (also known as Cinchona officianalis): Fainting or unconsciousness (syncope) after great loss of blood by mother during labor.

CICUTA: Spasmodic rigidity with jerking.

LAUROCERASUS: Asphyxia. Blue Face, gasping for breath or imperceptible breathing. Twitching in face.

LACHESIS: Blue face, cyanosis (also Laurocerasus).

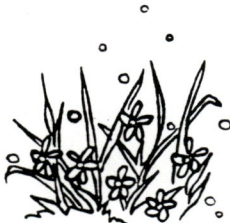

With infants, in emergency situations, the response should be almost immediate with the right remedy. If there is no change within one or at most two minutes, depending on the urgency of the situation, give the next possible remedy. I had a case of a baby born with his cord wrapped around his neck; he was quite blue all over. I gave Aconite and when no change was seen in about 30 seconds, I switched to Laurocerasus. Before I could barely register what was happening the child turned pink, even to its fingers. For situations like this one I prefer to use the 200C potency, or the 1M.

Unfortunately, one of our most important remedies for unconsciousness and coma, homeopathic Opium, is now off the American market due to the FDA. I mention this because you will see it in the books for ailments from fright, unconsciousness, and other symptoms. This is one of the big tragedies in American homeopathy, as many lives were saved with Opium in potency.

Remember, as in all remedy pictures, the patient does not need to exhibit all of the symptoms listed. If most of the keynotes are there, it's worth a try. Of course do all other reasonable things, including a call for help if it is indicated. While help is coming, use the appropriate remedies.

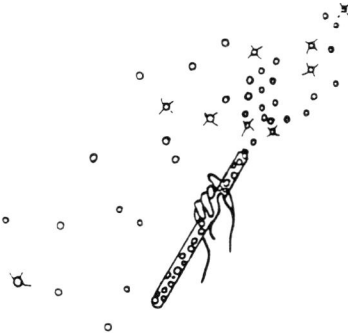

BIBLIOGRAPHY

Boericke, William M.D., *Materica Medica with Repertory*, 1982 reprint, B. Jain Publishers, New Delhi, India

Clark, John, *A Dictionary of Practical Materia Medica*, Vols. I, II, III, reprint 1984, B. Jain Publishers, New Delhi , India

Kent, J.T., M.D., *Lectures of Homeopathic Materia Medica*, 1904; and Repertory of Homeopathic Materia Medica, 1877, B. Jain Publishers, New Delhi, India

Yingling,W.A., M.D., *Accoucheur's Emergency Manual*, B. Jain Publishers, New Delhi, India

FURTHER BASIC BOOKS FOR THE HOME ABOUT HOMEOPATHY

Curing Colic and Lactose Intolerance With Homeopathy, Shiloh, Jana, M.A., Rocky Mountain Homeopathic Press, P.O. Box 10265, Sedona, AZ 86336 $4.95

A consise, practical guide for dealing with this very common malady of children.

Everybody's Guide to Homeopathic Medicines, Cummings, Stephan, F.N.P. and Ullman, Dana, M.P.H., J.P. Tarcher, 9110 Sunset Blvd., Los Angeles, CA 90069 $9.95

A good introductory book with practical information about acute health problems as well as the more common remedies that cure.

Homeopathic Medicine at Home, Panos, M., M.D., and Heimlich, J., 1980, J.P. Tarcher, 9110 Sunset Blvd., Los Angeles, CA 90069 $9.95

A good introduction with antecdotes about Dr. Panos' experiences with the remedies. Acute illness is emphasized as well as helpful charts for injuries and diseases.

Who is Your Doctor and Why, Shadman, Alonzo, M.D., 1958, Keats, New Canaan, CT - 1980 reprint. $3.95

This book was written by a surgeon-homeopath about his experiences. Included are useful guides on remedies for common ailments.

HOMEOPATHIC PHARMACIES

Dolisos Homeopathic Medicines
3014 Rigel Avenue
Las Vegas, NV 89102
1-800-824-8455

Boericke and Tafel
2381 Circadian Way
Santa Rosa, CA 95407
800-876-9505

Standard Homeopathic Pharmacy
P.O. Box 61067
Los Angeles, CA 90061
213-321-4284

Hahnemann Pharmacy
1918 Bonita Avenue
Berkeley, CA 94704
415-548-5015
This pharmacy rents birthing kits!

Boiron
1208 Amosland Road
P.O. Box 54
Norwood, PA 19074
800-258-8823

Some health food stores stock individual homeopathic remedies as well as books about homeopathy.

HOMEOPATHIC ORGANIZATIONS

Newsletters and information about homeopathic training are available from these organizations:

International Foundation
of Homeopathy
2366 Eastlake Avenue E. #301
Seattle, WA 98102
206-324-8230

National Center for Homeopathy
1500 Massachusetts, NW
Washington, D.C. 20005
703-548-7790

Pacific Academy of
Homeopathic Medicine
1678 Shattuck Ave., #42
Berkeley, CA 94709
415-549-3475

Complementary Medicine Assoc.
4649 E. Malvern
Tucson, Arizona 85711
602-323-6291

SOURCES FOR HOMEOPATHIC BOOKS

Homeopathic Ed. Services
2124 Kittredge Street
Berkeley, CA 94704
800-359-9051

Homeopathic Informational
Resources
Oneida River, Park Drive
Clay N.Y. 13041
800-289-4447

The Bodhi Tree Bookstore
8585 Melrose Ave
Los Angeles CA 90069
213-659-1733

The Minimum Price
808 Peace Portal Dr., Ste. AA-234
Blaine, WA 98230
800-663-8272

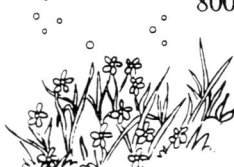

ABOUT THE AUTHOR

Jana Shiloh, M.A., has practiced homeopathy over the past ten years. She practiced extensively in India. She is presently committed to the grassroots development and education of homeopathy for those who recognize the advantages and limitations of allopathic medicine as it is today.

Ms. Shiloh is available to teach the following dynamic workshops in your community:

INTRODUCTION TO HOMEOPATHY: Family First Aid and Sports Medicine (Sports Medicine is optional)

ACUTE ILLNESSES AND HOMEOPATHIC TREATMENT FOR FAMILY USE

INTERMEDIATE SEMINAR IN ACUTE PRESCRIBING: Introducing Kent's Repertory

HOMEOPATHIC CASE TAKING

INTRODUCTION TO HOMEOPATHY AND MIDWIFERY

ACUTE PRESCRIBING IN MIDWIFERY

ELABORATIONS ON COLIC AND LACTOSE INTOLERANCE

For further information, write or call:

Jana Shiloh
Rocky Mountain Press
P.O. Box 10265
Sedona, AZ 86336
602-282-9362

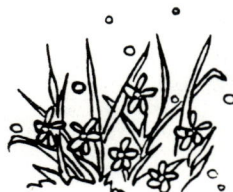